MARTIN

D1549774

GATEWAYS TO HEALTH

BUTTERFLY TAI CHI

HEALTH, ENERGY AND TRANQUILLITY IN TEN MINUTES A DAY

WATKINS PUBLISHING

LONDON

This edition published in the UK 2009 by
Watkins Publishing, Sixth Floor, Castle House,
75–76 Wells Street, London W1T 3QH

Conceived, created and designed by Duncan Baird Publishers

1 3 5 7 9 10 8 6 4 2

Designed by Clare Thorpe
Commissioned artwork by Conny Jude (www.connyjude.com)
and Art-4

Printed and bound in Great Britain

British Library Cataloguing-in-Publication Data Available

ISBN: 978-1-906787-19-6

www.watkinspublishing.co.uk

Contents

Introduction

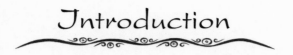

The Story of Tai Chi

Tai Chi Quian is one of the legendary arts of ancient China. There are many myths about its origins; the most popular and well known tells of its creation 800 years ago by Daoist master Zhang Sanfeng who lived in the Wudang Mountains. The story goes that he had dreams in which the secrets of Tai Chi were taught to him and that, using these dreams as inspiration, he softened Kung Fu into a more spiritually focused martial art.

However, the earliest historical records we have of Tai Chi are only 300 years old and suggest that it was first developed in Chen village in Wenxian County in the Henan Province. It was practised by an army garrison commander and great warrior called Chen Wing Ting.

Many martial arts had developed throughout China due to many years of foreign invasions and peasant uprisings. But while previous arts had consisted of powerful quick movements, Tai Chi emphasized using the opponents' force against them: 'overcoming the vigorous with the soft', using 'one pound of weight to redirect 1000 pounds' and most of all 'adapting oneself to the opponent'. The Tai Chi movements from this period have both soft and gentle movements and energetic forceful strikes. As time went on Tai Chi continued to evolve away from its martial roots and the movements became far gentler and more health focused.

Many styles of Tai Chi developed throughout China and five main styles remain to this day: *Chen* (the original martial style); *Yang* (a softer, more circular form); *Wu* (known for its smaller stances and smaller movement); and second styles, another also named *Wu* (known for its quick short range movements); and *Sun* (known for its fast pace and advanced footwork).

The Tao

Tai Chi is an art drawn from the Chinese spiritual tradition known as Taoism (道). Taoism is over two thousand years old and translates into English as the 'Path', or the 'Way' and is more of a way of life or a spiritual path than a religion in the Western sense. Taoism is guided by The Three Jewels of the Tao; these are compassion, moderation and humility. Generally speaking, Taoist philosophy focuses on achieving harmony, health, longevity, immortality, spontaneity and effortless action (*wu wei*). Central to the Taoist philosophy is a belief in the underlying force or guiding principle in the universe called the Tao.

Tao is everything that is natural: all the laws of physics, the laws of science, the way your mind works, the rules of nature and biology. It affects everything: every plant, every animal and every person. In other words, Tao is the guiding force behind existence. In truth, Tao is not something that can be defined, it can only be experienced.

The aim of Taoism is to become at one with

Tao: to live in harmony with the fundamental structure and natural order of everything. This is not achieved through struggle but through going with the flow. If you resist you become a blockage in the natural order. By relaxing you become far more powerful. The great Tai Chi masters of old used to say, 'Water is the softest thing; because of its softness not even a tiger can hurt it with its claws, and it can wear through the hardest rock.'

In other words, always swim with the flow of the river. Tai Chi follows all these principles, and through relaxed Tai Chi practice it will become possible for you to experience the Tao.

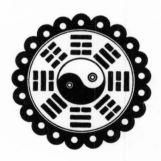

About Butterfly Tai Chi

The traditional styles of Tai Chi consist of a set of movements joined together like a slow dance, with one move flowing to another without hesitation. The form appears to the onlooker to be like clouds floating across the sky, or similar to a snake moving slowly along the floor. Each traditional form consists of 108 movements and really needs to be performed in a large hall or outside. The whole form can take over half an hour to finish.

In recent times it has become increasingly difficult for people to find room to practise such a long form and many find it hard to remember all the movements. So in the last 50 years shorter forms of Tai Chi have developed, the most popular being the '24 Move Form', a simplified form developed by Li Tian Ji.

I began to realize, though, that many of my students found

that even this form was hard to practise in a modern Western domestic setting, so I resolved to develop a form of Tai Chi that could be practised while standing on the spot. In a hotel room, for example, or by someone with restricted living space. However, in Tai Chi movement is required to keep the internal energy, or force, flowing and movements practised in a stationary position can lead to stagnation of the energy. I tried in vain to find a way to develop a form that would involve virtually no movement while maintaining the flow of Tai Chi, and I had all but given up when inspiration came from the most unlikely of places.

I noticed a butterfly moving its wings to warm itself in the sunshine and as I watched it occurred to me that this was one of the only animals I had ever seen exercise. Butterflies are cold-blooded and they flap their wings in the sunlight because they need to warm up a little before they can fly. The butterfly was stationary but inside everything was moving. By flapping its wings it was circulating the newly warmed blood throughout its being.

I suddenly knew where I was going wrong: if the practitioner was going to be stationary then the flow had to happen internally. I would design the Tai Chi movements so that they naturally enhanced the *Qi* flow in the order dictated by Chinese medicine. Thus, with the aid of my instructor, was born the Tai Chi set that is described in this book, one which I believe to be even more effective than the traditional Tai Chi forms as far as health benefits are concerned.

What are the Health Benefits of Tai Chi?

Tai Chi Quian is a traditional Chinese system of health preservation and illness prevention. Tai Chi could be seen as the healthiest art in existence as it includes the health benefits of calm and gentle exercise, along with the physiological and stress-relieving benefits of meditation and the curative power of acupuncture. For this reason, Tai Chi is frequently prescribed in China as a treatment for illnesses as diverse as high blood pressure, neurasthenia, pulmonary tuberculosis, nervous breakdown, impotence, anxiety disorder, depression, arthritis and even diabetes. The real power of Tai Chi, however, lies in its power to prevent illness.

Studies into the effects of Tai Chi have shown that despite the fact that the exercises are gentle and require relaxation, they also involve focus and visualization. They bring about great benefits to the functioning of the central nervous system while at the same time stimulating the cerebral cortex, causing stimulation in certain areas and offering protection in others. This allows the cerebral cortex to take a rest from any pathological excitement caused by mental diseases.

The meditative nature of the exercises brings about a relaxation response in the whole body and this has been proven to lower blood pressure and completely counteract the negative effects of stress. It has also been shown that those who practise Tai Chi are more calm and balanced during everyday life.

Disease prevention studies have revealed that those who practise Tai Chi have stronger muscles and bones, far more efficient cardiovascular, respiratory and metabolic systems, and lower blood pressure and cholesterol than non-practitioners. There is also evidence that Tai Chi enhances the regulatory functions of the central nervous system and the coordination of internal organs.

But there may be another hidden benefit to Tai Chi practice not yet known to science. Traditional Chinese medicine asserts that the body has natural patterns of an energy called *Qi* – also spelt 'chi', or in romanized Japanese, 'Ki'. The concept of *Qi* is fundamental to traditional Chinese culture. It is a form of spiritual energy that is part of every living thing that exists. It is the life force or ether of the west. The energy regulates the body and keeps it healthy through a system of channels called 'meridians'. Tai Chi was designed to ensure the correct and healthy flow of Qi through the body, thereby revitalizing the tissues and organs.

Finally, everything should move in unison, your mind should guide your body and each movement should be generated from the hips. Your eyes, body, legs, arms and breathing should all be coordinated. You may find that your breathing becomes deeper and that you breathe more from your abdomen during your practice. This is of great benefit to your health and will develop naturally over time.

The movements are best practised in order but do feel free to practise each one in turn until you are comfortable with them. Remember, Tai Chi is about moving in a natural way so don't be too rigid with your movements. The human body has its own natural angles and your body is unique, so if you find performing a movement uncomfortable in the way I describe it adapt it for yourself. Take the time daily to practise them as an investment in yourself, preferably in a place free from distraction where you are unlikely to be disturbed. Above all things, relax and enjoy the exercises.

Yin and Yang

It's important when practising Tai Chi to understand the principle of yin and yang. Yin and yang represent the two opposites that exist in all things. The concept is usually expressed in a diagram known as the Tai Chi Symbol. The black side (yin) represents the dark, cold, destructive female force, and the white (yang) represents the light, warm, creative male force. These forces can be seen reflected in all things: night and day, sun and moon, male and female.

In Tai Chi we aim to achieve perfect balance through the harmony of opposites. Each Tai Chi movement contains a reflection of yin and yang. To truly master Tai Chi one must be able to achieve the balance of yin and yang not only in the practice of the Tai Chi movements but also in every aspect of one's life.

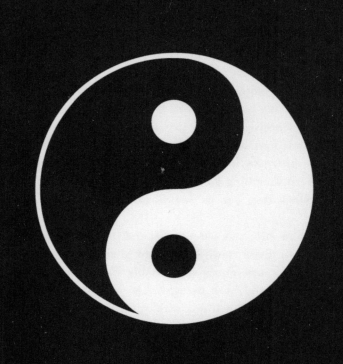

Butterfly Tai Chi Basic Set

Horse Riding Stance

All the exercises in this set are performed from a starting position called 'Horse Riding Stance'. This posture is used in virtually every Oriental martial art, and is often used as a separate exercise to increase one's leg strength, concentration, deep breathing and *Qi* flow. In Chinese, this is called '*Zhang Zong*' or 'standing like a tree'.

Stand with your feet parallel and shoulder-width apart. Bend your knees into a shallow squat, making sure you are comfortable. Keep your back straight and head upright. Let your arms hang in a relaxed manner with your fingers curled slightly inwards.

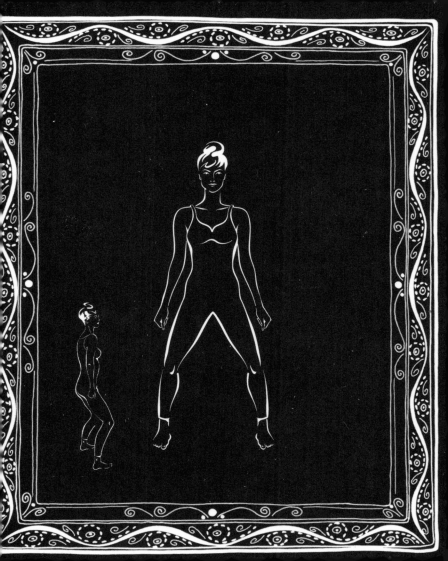

Lifting Water

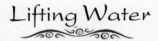

This should be done at the beginning of any set of exercises as an aid to calming the mind. Some people find it beneficial to imagine that their arms are being lifted as if floating on water.

Stand in the relaxed Horse Riding Stance with your hands at your sides. Inhale and lift your arms upwards in front of your body, keeping your wrists relaxed so your hands hang down, and your fingers slightly curled inwards. As you lift your arms, straighten your knees slightly so that your body rises in time with the arms' lifting motion. This exercise develops a sense of relaxed ease that ought to be maintained throughout all exercises.

Relax your arms and gradually let them return to their position on either side of your body. As you do this let your bodyweight naturally return you to the relaxed Horse Riding Stance.

Repeat 10 times.

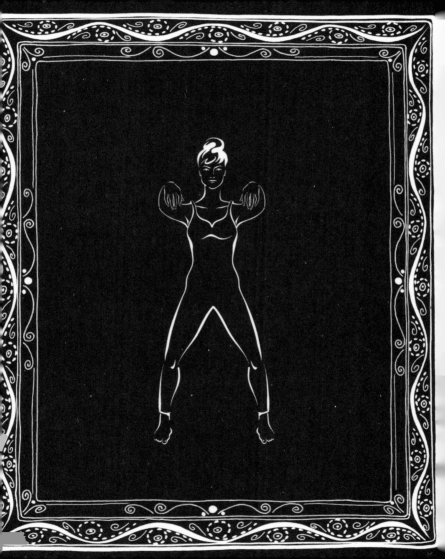

Pat the Horse

This exercise is for your *lungs*. The movement is named after the natural movement of running your hands though a horse's mane, but you may find it helpful to imagine the forceful breath of a horse and the strength the animal possesses.

1 Stand in the Horse Riding Stance. Take a deep breath and allow your ribcage to expand. As you breathe in, lift both your arms to your sides at shoulder height with your palms facing forward. Simultaneously turn your torso to the right. Turn your palms so that they both face upwards.

2 Bend your right arm at the elbow so that its palm faces forwards behind your head.

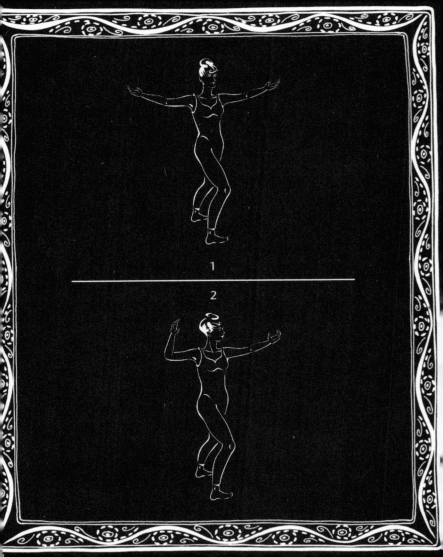

1

2

3   Exhale and start to rotate the torso back towards the left, turning your head with your body and keeping your gaze on your left hand. As you move, push forwards purposefully with your right palm whilst simultaneously pulling back with your left hand, palm still facing up. As the left hand moves to the left and the right comes back into view, move your focus onto your right hand.

4   Continue the turning motion to the left and let the hands' paths continue until you are able to turn your palms upwards to create the mirror of position 1. Right hand forwards and left hand back, now you can bend your left hand to face the palm forwards and repeat the 'push' motion on the other side.

Keep your focus on your lungs and project the force through your lungs as you exhale.

Repeat the sequence 5 times on each side.

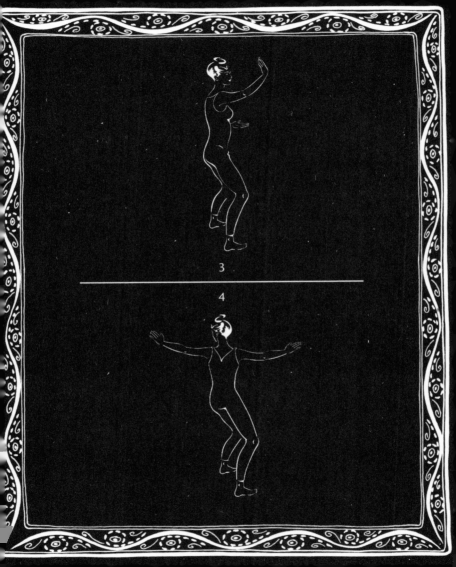

3

4

Needle at the Bottom of the Sea

This starts with the same movement as Pat the Horse, so links perfectly. When practising imagine that you are reaching down to pick up a needle from between your feet. The bend in this exercise brings healing and rejuvenation to your *kidneys*.

1   Take a deep breath, expanding your ribcage. Simultaneously turn your torso to the right and lift both arms out to your sides at shoulder height, palms facing up. Hold your hands with fingers together in a kind of 'karate chop' position.

2   In one flowing motion, bend your right arm, rotate your body to the left and bring the right hand past your head in a sweeping 'chopping' motion. The main movement should come from the rotation of your waist. Your eyes should follow the movement of your chopping hand, while the other hand should be kept out of the way.

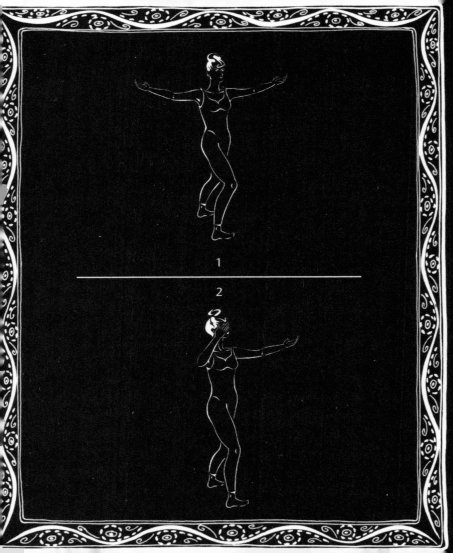

1

2

3 Keeping your eyes on your right hand, continue your chopping motion by bending at the waist and placing your right hand between your feet almost touching the ground. If your flexibility does not allow you to bend this far with comfort, slowly increase your range of motion as time goes on. As you bend over, remember to focus your mind on your kidneys.

As you return to an upright standing position you will notice that you are back in the start position and ready to repeat the movement on the other side by turning your torso to the left.

Repeat the sequence 5 times on each side.

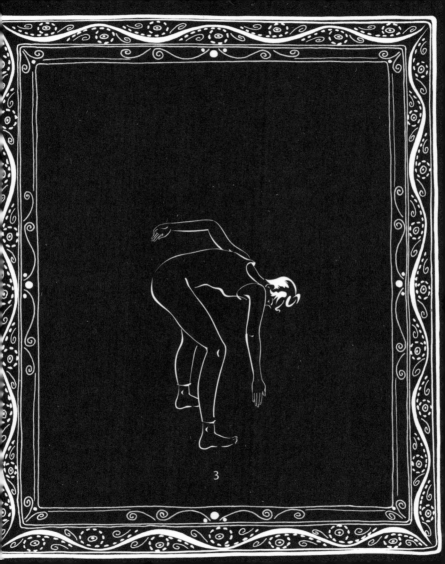

Golden Cockerel Stands On One Leg

～∽∾⌒∾∽～

You can flow on to this movement from your last 'Needle at the Bottom of the Sea' but to begin with you may like to start from a relaxed Horse Riding Stance. This movement, as the name suggests, imitates the movement of a cockerel. Make sure that your attention is on a rising, upwards movement. The force will naturally focus on your *liver*.

I Start this movement with an inhalation coordinated with lifting your right arm and your right leg at the same time. The lift of the arm comes from the shoulder and the leg lifts from the hip. The hand and foot are both relaxed. Your palm is kept face down. The other hand remains by your side with the hand at the level of the raised knee.

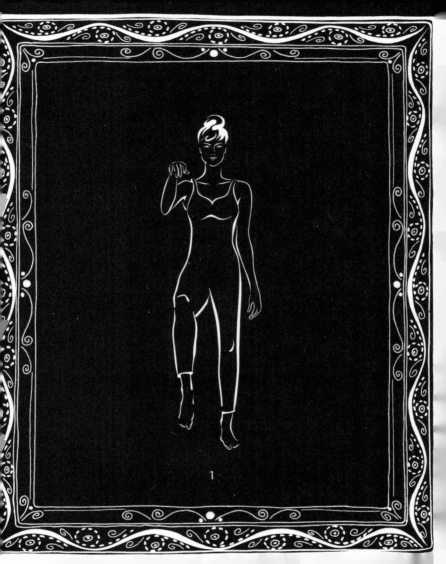

1

2   This move requires balance and focus. Once you have managed this small lift, work your way up until your thigh is just about parallel with the floor and your right hand is by your head, palm facing up. As you reach the top of the movement, remember to focus on your *liver*.

Exhale and gently lower your body back to the Horse Riding Stance, then repeat with the left arm and leg.

Repeat the sequence 5 times on each side.

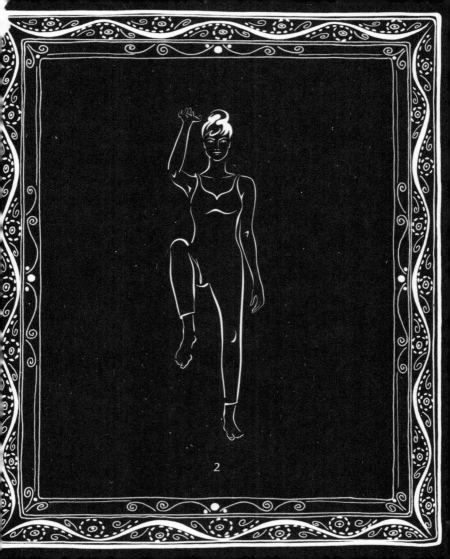

2

Opening the Rainbow

You can flow into this exercise from the last 'Golden Cockerel' exercise or just start from a Horse Riding Stance. This exercise is named after the rainbow which has an association with happiness in all cultures. The focus on the movement is the *heart*. A healthy heart will lead to a happy life.

1 Standing in Horse Riding Stance, bring the backs of your hands together at groin level.

2 As you inhale, lift both hands in a relaxed fashion in front of your body, elbows bent and pointing away from your body, and palms facing down with the backs of the hands touching slightly at chest level.

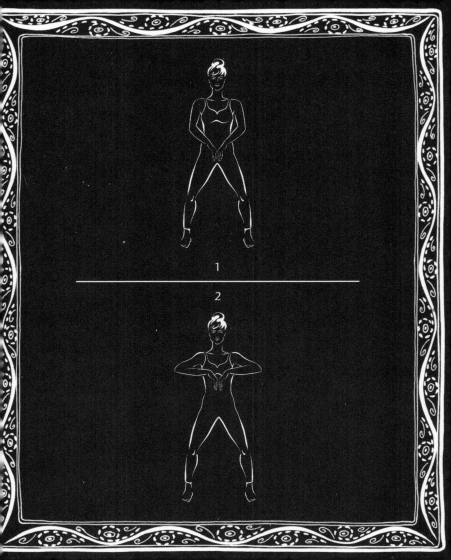

3 Lift hands and bring arms out to the sides, palms turning up, whilst simultaneously bending backwards so that there is a gentle curve in your back. Look upwards and expand your hands outwards so that they too face the sky, palms facing up, and exhale.

When you have finished exhaling, reverse your movements, bringing your hands back in front of you and straightening your back. Lower your hands until you are back in the start position.

Repeat the sequence 5 times.

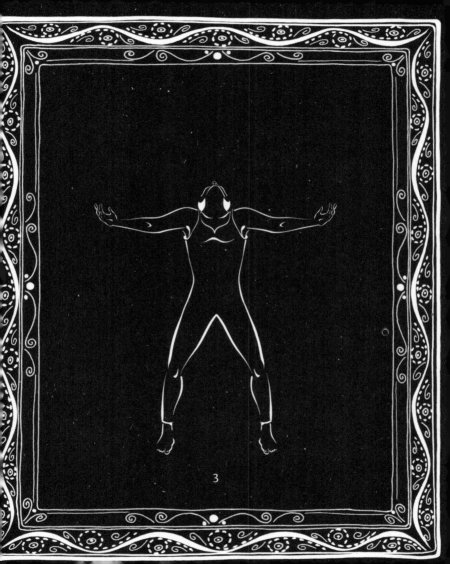

3

Cow Turns to
Look at the Moon

As with all exercises in this set you can easily link this to the last exercise. In China the cow is a symbol of abundance and wealth. The cow is also known for its amazingly efficient digestive system so it is no coincidence that the focus of this exercise is the *stomach* and *digestive system*.

1   On the final rainbow exercise, don't bring your arms all the way back down but simply turn the hands to face each other at chest height. Wrists should be bent and fingers pointing towards each other as if holding a ball. In Tai Chi we call this the 'ball holding' position. If you are starting this exercise from a relaxed Horse Riding Stance, simply lift your hands into this position.

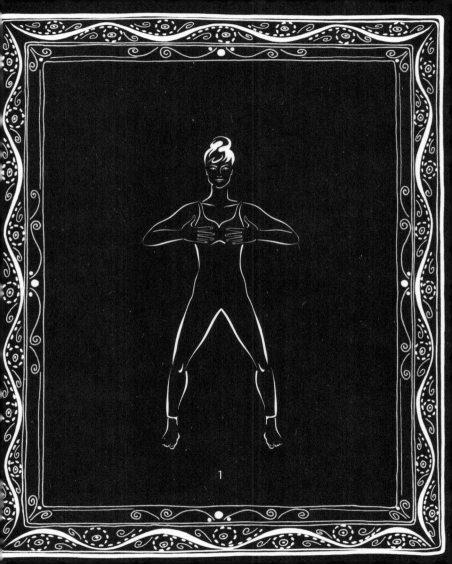

1

2   Exhale and turn to the right from the waist. As
    you do so, keep your hands in the ball holding
    position. Continue turning as far as you can
    without moving your foot position. With practice,
    you will find that you are looking directly behind
    you. When you reach the maximum range of your
    motion, turn your palms to face outwards.

    Inhale and return to your starting position,
    turning your hands back to the ball holding
    position as you go. Turn to the left and repeat
    movement on the other side.

    Repeat sequence 5 times on each side. Make sure
    you keep your focus on your *digestive system*.

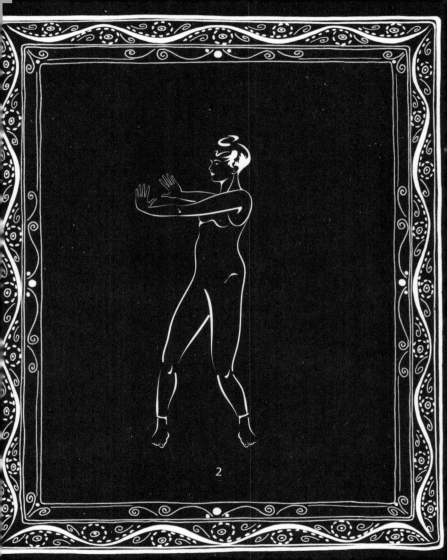

2

Closing the Door

This final exercise is used to bring all the forces of the body into harmony and balance. In China it is performed after any form of spiritual exercise or even just when you need to feel balanced. This exercise works by leading the *Qi* down through the body in an equal fashion and thus harmonizing the whole of your being.

1   Stand in Horse Riding Stance. Breathe slowly and deeply, and calm your mind. Inhale and turn your palms outwards and upwards, lifting and opening both arms in one flowing movement until they reach shoulder level.

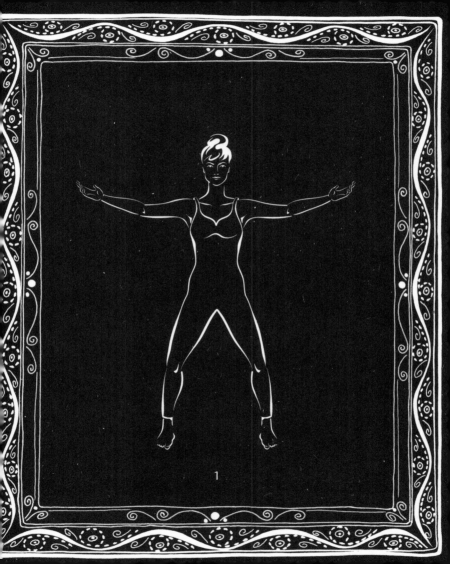

1

2 As your hands reach shoulder height inhale, bend your arms upwards at the elbow and turn your hands to face palm downwards, moving them down past your face and head.

3 Continue to move your arms downwards, letting every part of your being relax until your hands are at waist height.

Each time you complete any future sets of exercises you should end with this exercise. One or two repetitions will normally be enough.

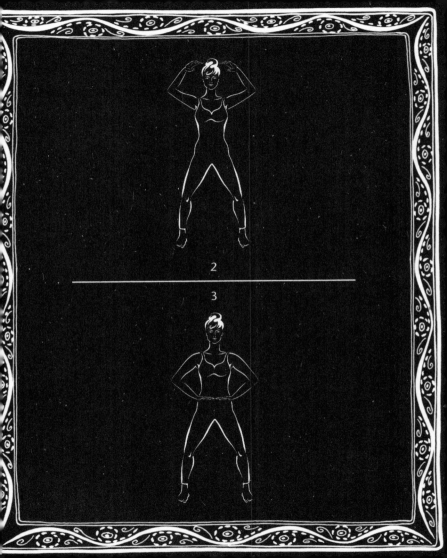

2

3

Butterfly Tai Chi Advanced Set

This set is for those who have already mastered the first set of Tai Chi exercises and would like to move on to something more advanced and challenging. Like the basic set, the advanced set consists of five exercises. Although not pictured here you should start with the opening (Lifting Water) and closing (Closing the Door) exercises as taught in the previous set. These exercises are more strenuous and involve dynamic movements and kicking movements that are more challenging than the previous set.

As before, the exercises start from the Horse Riding Stance. However, in this set you should lower your stance with feet further apart and form clenched fists with palms facing upwards and held at the hips. Remember to keep your back straight and head upright and most of all remember to keep relaxed and focused.

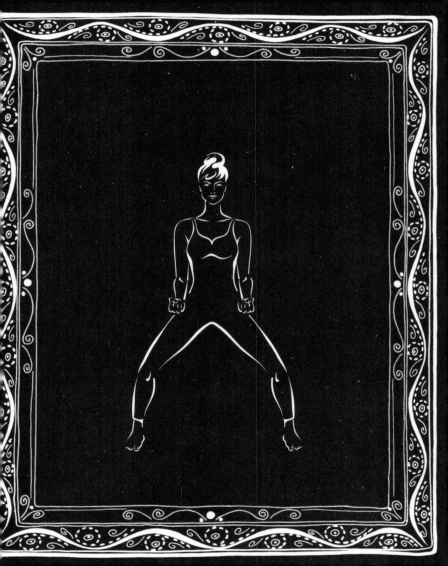

Alternate Punching

We start this set with a very forceful exercise. The movement is made one hand at a time, starting with your right hand. Each punch should be coordinated with a forceful exhalation. The breath should be forceful but the punch should be gentle. The focus of this exercise is the *lungs*.

1   Stand in a deep Horse Riding Stance with fists clenched, palms up at hip level. Take a deep breath. As you exhale move your right fist forwards from the hip, rotating your hand inwards so that your clenched fist is palm down. Don't extend your arm fully but rather leave a small bend in your elbow. Simultaneously, pull your left arm back, palm up. The whole movement should be flowing.

2   Reverse this process to return your arm to starting position. Repeat on the other side.

Repeat the sequence 10 times on each side.

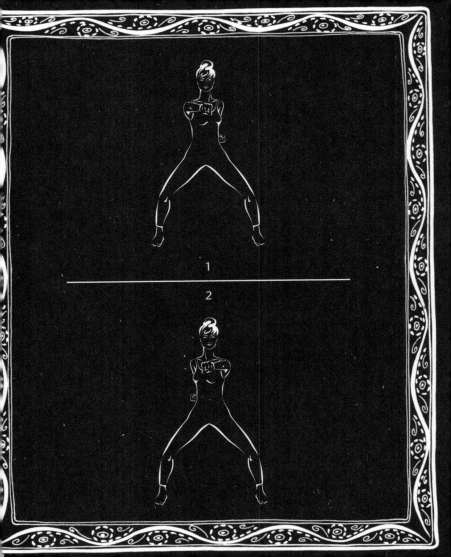

1

2

Dredging the Sea and Looking at the Sky

This exercise involves a lot of movement so you may have to relax your Horse Riding Stance a little and allow for a small pivot of the feet. As with the Needle at the Bottom of the Sea exercise in the last set, the bending in this exercise causes the force to gather in the *kidneys*.

1 Take a deep breath and allow your ribcage to expand. Simultaneously turn your torso slightly to the right. As you do this, bend forwards slightly and thrust both hands out and down, opening your fists and crossing your hands just in front of your right knee.

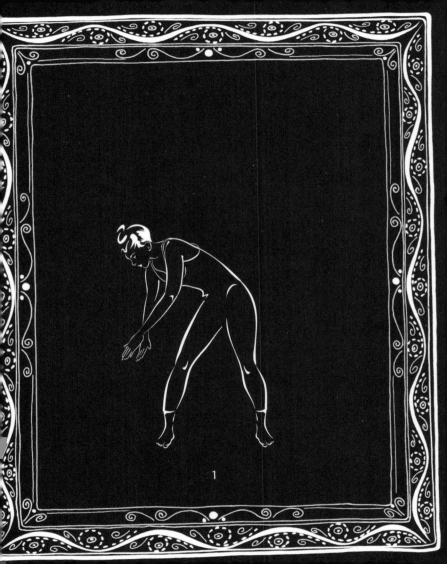

1

2 Taking a deep breath, straighten up and lift both your gently extended arms with your wrists still crossed high in the air. Keep your gaze on your crossed hands throughout.

3 As you exhale, rotate your waist to the left and gently lower your arms to bring them both, still crossed, in front of your left knee.

Repeat the sequence 10 times on each side.

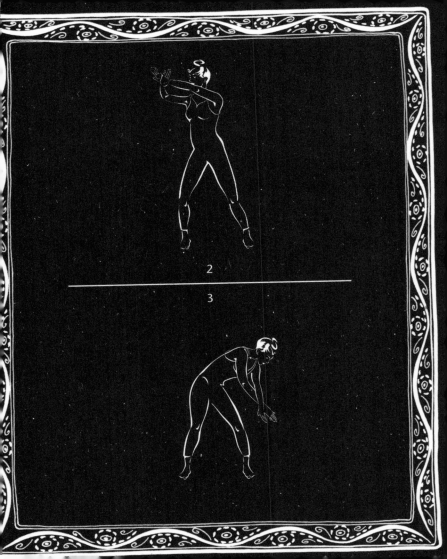

2

3

Push Kick

You can flow on to this movement from the last, but to begin with you may like to start from a relaxed Horse Riding Stance. This movement, like the Golden Cockerel, should focus on an upwards movement to aid the *liver*.

I Start this movement with an inhalation coordinated with lifting your arms and your right leg at the same time. The hands are crossed, palms facing the front of the body with the right hand in front of the left, knee bent and hip turned out at 45 degrees.

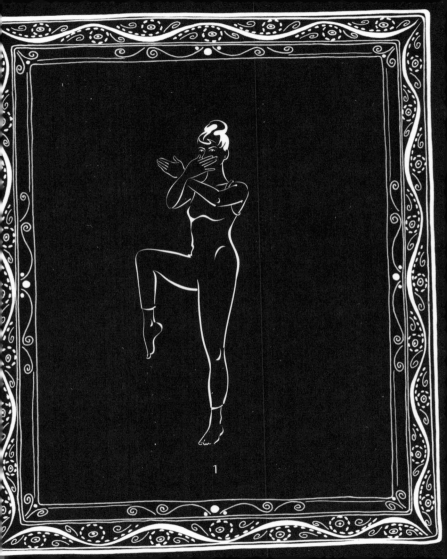

1

2 As you exhale, kick outwards with the bottom of your raised right foot as if pushing something with the sole of your foot; at the same time push out both hands, palms facing out. The right hand is above the kicking leg, the left mirrors it on the other side.

Reverse your movements to gently lower your body back to the Horse Riding Stance, then repeat with the left leg.

Repeat the sequence 10 times on each side.

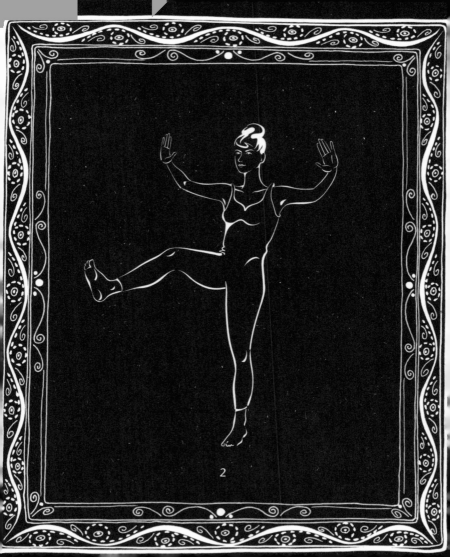

2

Opening the Chest

In this exercise we focus on the *heart*. Like the Opening the Rainbow movement, this exercise works by stretching the chest and expanding the ribcage. It's important in this exercise to be gentle but also to get a good range of movement.

1   Standing in a deep Horse Riding Stance, bring your hands together in front of your body at chest level, wrists bent and fingers pointing towards each other in 'ball holding' position.

2   As you inhale, lift and extend your arms backwards as if they are two doors opening outwards. This should be done in a calm, relaxed way. Continue this until you reach your maximum stretch and then return your hands to your front.

Repeat 10 times.

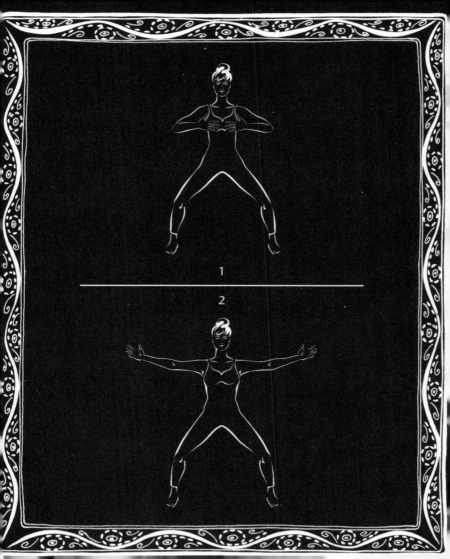

1

2

Double Dragons
Spiralling on the Pillar

As with all exercises in this set you can easily link this to the last exercise. In this exercise your body is the pillar and your arms are the twin dragons rotating around your torso. This exercise brings health to your *stomach* and *digestive system*.

1 Stand in a relaxed Horse Riding Stance and take a deep breath. Exhale and straighten your knees, turning your body slightly to the right while simultaneously bringing your left hand up from your hip and moving it to waist height across the front of your body. At the same time, do the opposite with your right arm: keeping your fist clenched, bring the arm behind you, with the back of your hand facing your lower back.

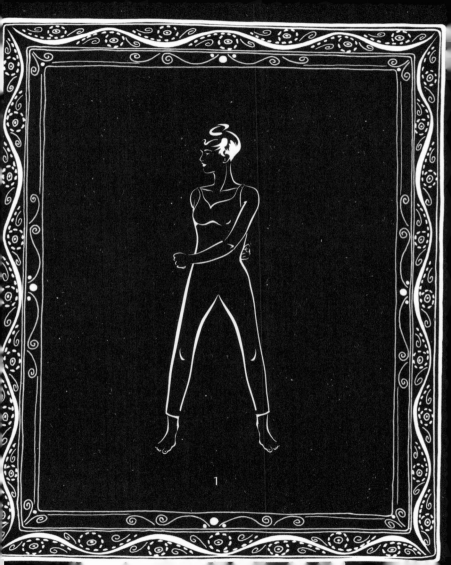

1

2   Continue turning as far as you can without moving your foot position. As you reach the maximum range of your motion, swing your body weight at your knees and start to turn your body back to the left. As you turn to the left your hands need to swap positions: in one coordinated, flowing movement bring your right fist from behind your back to your front and move your left hand with the flow of the turning movement to end up behind your back.

Repeat the sequence 10 times on each side.

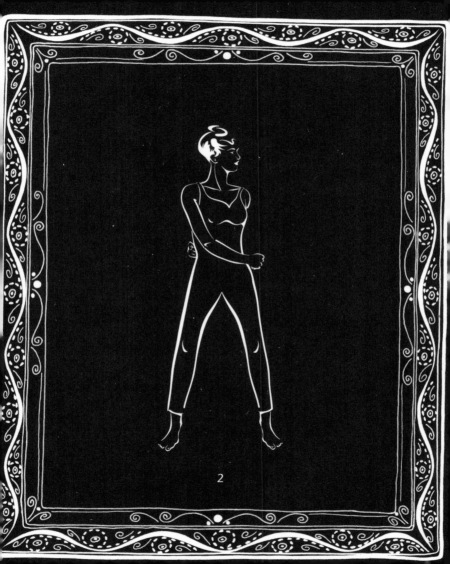

2

Acknowledgements

Dedicated with the upmost respect to my teacher
Bo Ou Mander.

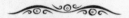